O RHD NEGATIVE (O-) BLOODTYPE AND CATAMENIAL ENDOMETRIOSIS

CATAMENIAL BLOOD

THEORIES INCLUDE MEN

BY

GLYNIS D. WALLACE D.M.D.

ISBN-13: 978-1533641991

ISBN-10: 1533641994

DEDICATION

I dedicate this book to all fighting and surviving the life trials of catamenial endometriosis.

In times of change, learners inherit the earth, while the learned find themselves beautifully equipped to deal with a world that no longer exists.

ERIC HOFFER

But they that wait upon the Lord shall renew their strength; they shall mount up with wings as eagles; they shall run, and not be weary, and they shall walk, and not faint.

ISAIAH 40 1:3

Contents

CHAPTER 5   45

FOODS TO AVOID

INTRODUCTION

My first book Living with Lung and Colon Endometriosis: Catamenial Pneumothorax describes my maze-like healthcare journey. It served to help educate a global patient and provider community to better understand the prevalence, hardship and current treatment options for this benign destructive disease with no cure. I was hopeful it would create global understanding among a cross section of medical specialties, ultimately leading to quicker, easier, less invasive test for widespread global diagnosis, and subsequent treatment regimes.

Endometriosis has been diagnosed and documented in the male urinary system.

This book serves to alert the global community to a possible connection between Rhesus D-negative blood and Catamenial Endometriosis. Many are familiar with blood groups O, A, B, AB and know their blood type, but have no idea about the other component Rhesus D- negative or positive due to the presence or absence of inherited rhesus factor on the surface of red blood cells. This is extremely important especially in women's health during childbearing and lifesaving blood transfusions. While researching many of nature's medicines to restore my health and enhance the healing process, an unmistakable eerie similarity between foods to avoid for endometriosis and Rh negative was illuminated.

Endometriosis refers to displaced tissue from the mucous membrane of the uterus where females carry their babies. Endometrial cells on my lung and colon were not attached to the reproductive system confirmed at diagnosis. Where are the endometrial cells in men traveling from? Answers to this question may be the first steps to a cure.

Catamenial pneumothorax is referred to as menstrual lung collapse, blood in a place air is supposed to be; endometrial implants appear on the lung like a chocolate cyst and release blood between the lung and its lining known as the pleura. Catamenial - of or relating to menstruation or the "menstrual period" and Pneumothorax - lung collapse.

There are five presentations of endometriosis in the chest referred to as Thoracic Endometriosis Syndrome, which is life threatening and can be fatal. My story, as well as other presentations and theories of endometrial cell migration, discussed.

CHAPTER 1
CATAMENIAL ENDOMETRIOSIS

Statistics reveal over 176 million women and undetermined numbers of men globally have this benign non-cancerous destructive disease endometriosis, defined as endometrial cells which line the uterus in females, travel outside attaching to other body organs. Of course, this definition will have to be changed to include males. The cells bleed every month in response to the hormonal, catamenial (cat-a-me-ni-al) monthly menstrual cycle.

Remember the old joke in reference to the probable cause. Career woman's disease, strong X-chromosome liberated cells. Well endometriosis is no joke, I'm bloody serious, although it may not be a death sentence in most cases, it is a life sentence and with lung involvement, Catamenial pneumothorax can quickly become a medical emergency. Blood in a place air is supposed to be leading to menstrual lung collapse results in the inability to breathe.

Endometriosis is estrogen driven, so what does this mean? To treat the disease and keep endometriosis under control, you must control estrogen and during that time, you will not be able to get into your favorite tight jeans.

Your breast may feel enlarged generating sensitivity, and I cannot decide if this is a benefit or not. You are more assertive, less patient and hot when everyone else is cold. There are many pharmaceuticals with a few side effects, to aid in estrogen suppression. You can ask your physician to give you a breakdown of those currently on the market. Diet change is also highly recommended and essential for favorable long-term outcomes. There are estrogen-containing foods and estrogen inhibiting foods. Also, foods to avoid which parallel Rh- negative recommendations. Diet control is extremely important because estrogen gets trapped and lingers in fat cells also waiting for a turn to enter the catamenial hormonal party.

Catamenial endometriosis found in almost every body organ, cause unusual symptoms periodically occur. No matter where it is located, endometriosis is a Gynecology disease with secondary Pulmonary, Cardiothoracic, Neurology, Gastroenterology, Colorectal, Urology, Nephrology, Ophthalmology, Orthopedic, Dermatology, ENT symptoms. Every medical specialty should add endometriosis to their differential diagnosis. When perplexing things happen monthly, you just cannot explain, and you are pressed for answers reply, "I think it's Catamenial."

Pelvic pre-menstrual syndrome has been recognized for years. What expressions exist for endometrial cells in other areas of the body?

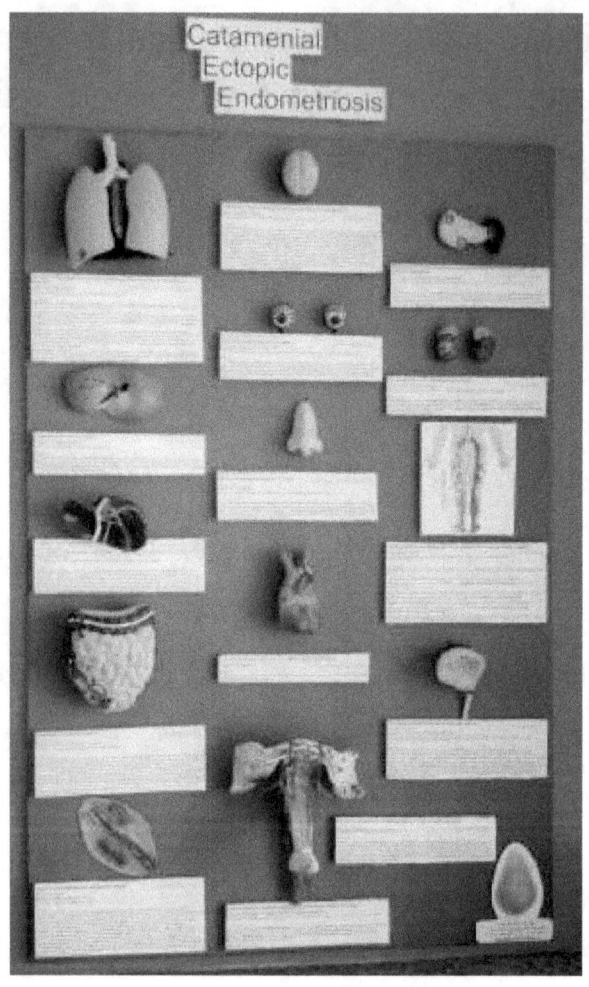

(See reference section)

CATAMENIAL LUNG

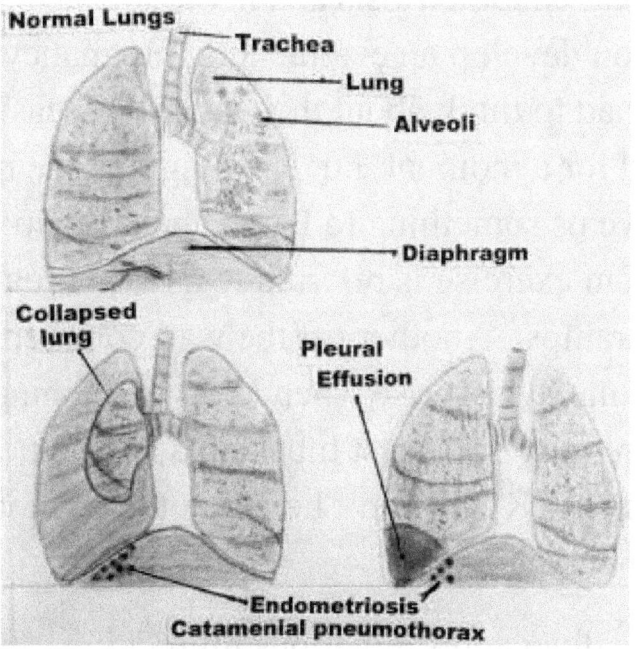

I became cynical after my close brushes with death and annoying recurrent lung collapses but quickly redeveloped a much needed sense of humor required to overcome and rise above obstacles and stigma.

A comical memory of the time I was explaining the weird complications associated with lung endometriosis and my associate asked: "can you develop an ectopic lung pregnancy"? I really had to think about the way this disease is viewed for a moment, but it did lighten the mood and give us something to laugh about. Pain in my side from exercise is referred to as menstrual chest cramps. Another off the wall comment caught me by surprise when I was explaining blood removal by chest tube and a colleague blurted out "Kotex can't help you there," and now they are taxed.

Five diverse presentations mimicking other diseases can manifest with endometriosis within the chest delaying diagnosis.

They are collectively referred to as Thoracic Endometriosis Syndrome.

Symptoms:

Most relevant and noticeable: radiating Catamenial pain in the shoulder from fluid causing pleurisy near the diaphragm. Becomes more severe with breathing, coughing or sneezing

Chest pain

Shortness of breath

Coughing, severe with direct air blowing from a fan or other sources

Coughing up or tasting blood

Crackling or wheezing

A feeling under the skin in the chest sometimes described as a "bubbling sensation" by many women

CATAMENIAL HEMOTHORAX

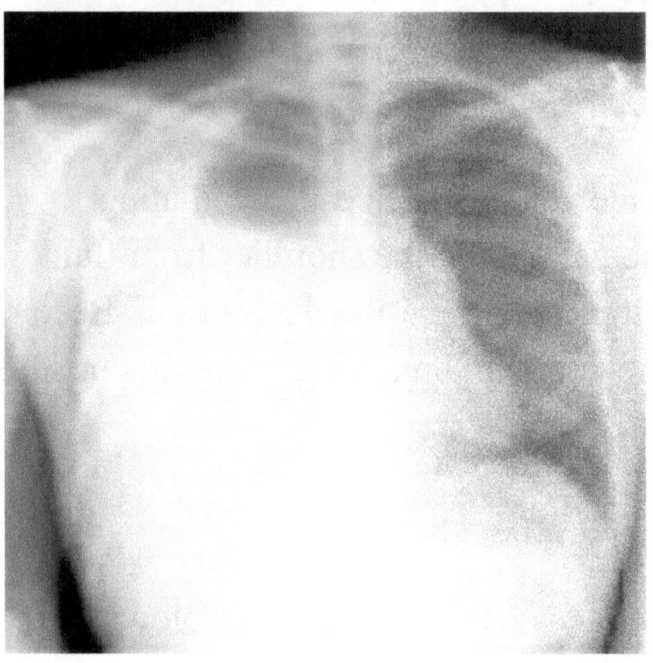

Blood fills the space between the lung and its lining the pleura. This was my first presentation. I had 3400 cc of blood on my right lung. There was no way of knowing how long blood had been accumulating monthly. The body will resorb it in small amounts without surgical intervention found out later.

A slight pain on the lower right side especially after running produced most of my discomfort. If any air blew on me from a fan or air conditioner, a violent coughing episode would occur, which I found extremely embarrassing as watery eyes developed disrupting any activity I was involved in, to include treating patients. Coughing became more frequent, and I had initially associated with allergies due to my recent move to Texas. There was no reason to suspect fluid on my lung or any other serious complication. Pain on the right side was mild, tolerable and I was hoping it was gallstones or something simple requiring non-invasive treatment. A strange phenomenon, my mother, knew something was seriously wrong long before diagnosis, and felt there was swelling on the right side of my face, which appeared normal in my eyes maybe due to slow accumulation. Plus who could have ever imagined accommodating large amounts of blood in the chest Physicians treating me were shocked wondering how it got there without any trauma.

11

Endometriosis in the chest is still under recognized and under diagnosed, but so much more is known about it.

CATAMENIAL PNEUMOTHORAX

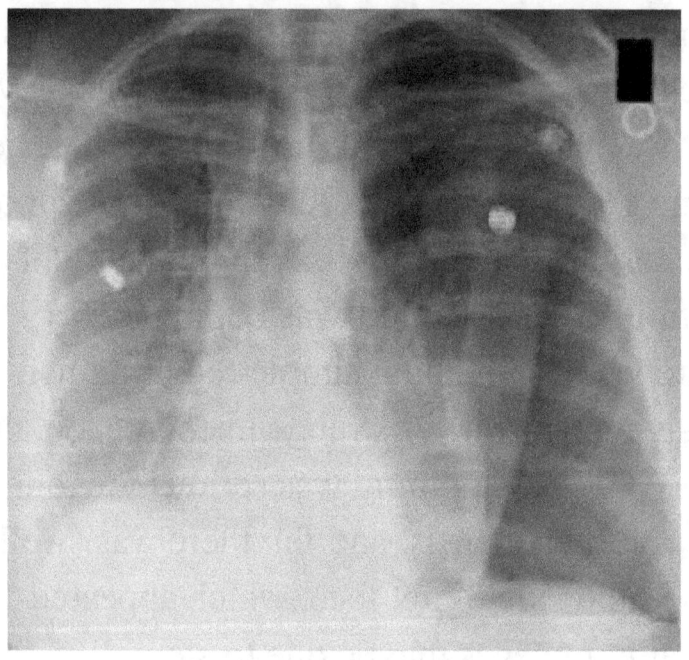

Lung collapse with active endometrial cells located between the lung and its lining the pleura, with air moving in by an unknown mechanism through fenestrations in the diaphragm

CATAMENIAL HEMOPNEUMOTHORAX

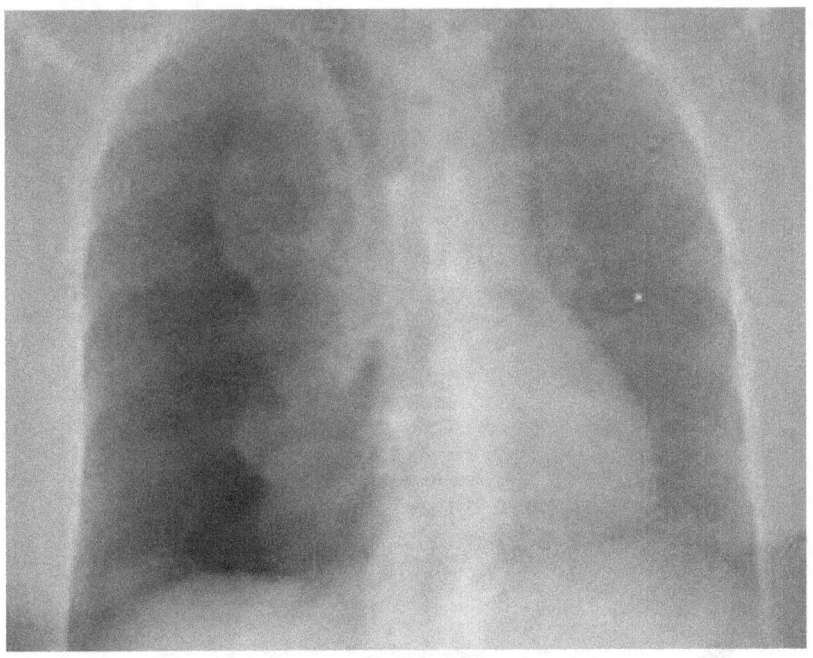

A combination of two conditions air and blood is present in the chest cavity, thus the lung cannot expand. This can lead to a tension pneumothorax which I experienced in 2002. The affected lung, which has a great deal of elastic tissue, shrivels affecting the unaffected side of the chest. This causes compression of the opposite lung which can compromise the return flow of blood to the heart, quickly becoming a life-threatening medical emergency. Yes, you can die from endometriosis.

CATAMENIAL HEMOPTYSIS

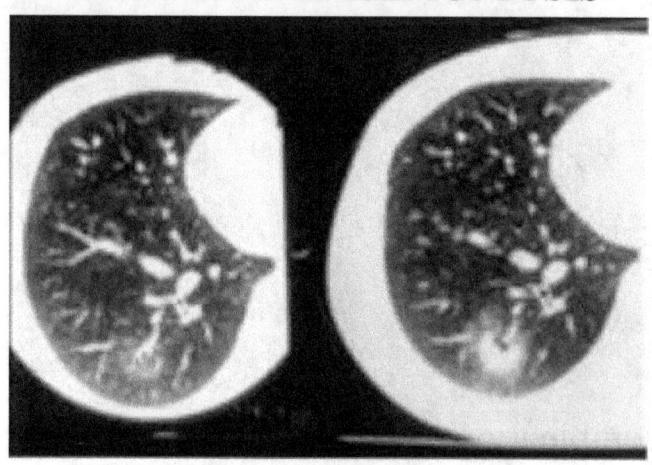

Before menses **During menses**

Endometrial cells are located in the tracheobronchial tree. Cat scan should be taken during menses to assist diagnosis.

Chest x-rays appear normal. Patients taste or cough up a teaspoon to one cup of blood monthly and tend to be younger as compared to other patients with thoracic endometriosis syndrome. It is recurrent monthly coinciding with menses.

ENDOMETRIOSIS LUNG NODULES

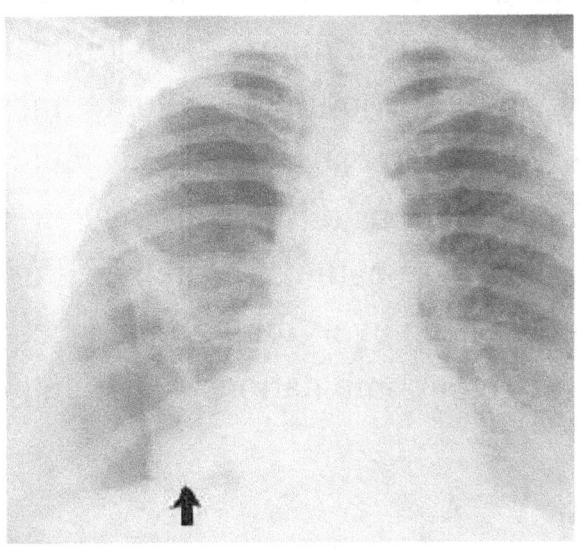

Endometriosis lung nodules: Many women have no symptoms at all. Nodules are found on a chest x-ray, cat-scan or MRI.

Surgeons narrative summaries of treatment included in the book "Living with Lung and Colon Endometriosis: Catamenial Pneumothorax".

OTHER CATAMENIAL ORGANS

CATAMENIAL COLON

Symptoms include gas pain with pressure, bloating, constipation, diarrhea, abdominal cramping, nausea, vomiting and sometimes rectal bleeding. During my surgery, the distal transverse and ileocecal sections of the colon were removed. The colon is where natures medicines if used properly, will keep everything in balance. Finding the right combinations is difficult.

CATAMENIAL BLADDER

Symptoms include bloody urine during menses with painful and more frequent urination. My colon endometriosis was attached to the outside of my bladder but did not invade. Urology found an indentation from a mass poking in from the back of the bladder during a cystoscopy.

CATAMENIAL BRAIN

Symptoms include severe headaches during menses, seizures and migraines. There is extensive research in this area. My mother who encouraged me to write my first book suffered from catamenial migraines. Driving into work, she would have to pull to the side of the road and her only relief was during pregnancy.

Maybe that was the reason she had nine children. Another family member suffered from catamenial seizures. I remember a tortuous time in between her first and second son when the monthly seizures caused great disturbances and inhibited her quality of life. There were periods when she could not drive or suffered humiliation of seizures occurring at work. Fortunately, she worked in a medical office with compassion, tolerance and understanding of the situation. But still it took a toll on her quality of life. After her second son, birth control pills controlled the seizures, until a hysterectomy and divine healing at age 40 occurred.

CATAMENIAL DIAPHRAGM

Includes symptoms of shoulder pain and fenestrations in diaphragmatic endometriosis allow air and gas in into chest resulting in recurrent catamenial Pneumothoraces

CATAMENIAL EYES

This is from endometriosis in the nasolacrimal duct, causing tears of blood monthly. This is probably the rarest form of Catamenial Endometriosis. I read a story about a girl from India, who was thought to possess special spiritual healing power because of this.

CATAMENIAL HEART

Symptoms include mild to severe chest pain and rapid, irregular heartbeat. I received three emails from women with endometriosis attached to their heart and put out a press release in 2007 to alert the global community titled Blog Debuts for Valentine's Day with 'Can Endometriosis Travel to the Heart?' — Yes, Says Dr. Wallace, Author, 'Living With Lung and Colon Endometriosis: Catamenial Pneumothorax.'

CATAMENIAL KIDNEYS

Obstruction of the ureter can cause severe lower back pain.

CATAMENIAL LIVER

Symptoms include cyst in the liver and severe right quadrant monthly epigastric pain. I have a small cyst in my liver that has not changed in 20 years, possibly hepatic endometrioma.

CATAMENIAL NOSE

Symptoms include monthly cyclic nose bleeds during menses, indicating ectopic endometrial tissue in the nasal cavity.

CATAMENIAL PANCREAS

Symptoms present similar to acute pancreatitis with severe abdominal pain.

CATAMENIAL PELVIC ENDOMETRIOSIS
Symptoms include heavy and irregular menses with mild to severe pain, infertility, and painful intercourse.

CATAMENIAL SCIATIC NERVE
Symptoms include pain radiation from the lower back down the back of the leg.

CATAMENIAL SKIN
Small nodules appear on the skin that become moist or bleed monthly. Endometrial cells can also move into healed scars from surgeries and respond to the hormonal cycle.

Endometriosis Confirmed in Men

Undetermined numbers of men have been diagnosed with endometriosis, presenting with symptoms of severe lower abdominal pain. Endometrioma of the abdominal wall, bladder, prostate and testicular endometriosis, have been reported.

GYN Oncology found no endometriosis attached to the reproductive system during my first surgery for diagnosis, confirmation and removal of tumor masses attached to the colon. This initiated more questions than answers as to how endometrial cells migrated to the colon and lung, which is still an unresolved mystery.

Ninety percent of the women, who write me with endometriosis in the chest, have children. They had no problems conceiving or with infertility and symptoms became evident years after childbearing.

Maybe catamenial endometriosis in men will provide some answers. "Tissue is the Issue."

There is currently no cure for endometriosis!

Chapter 2
O Rhesus D Negative Blood

RhD negative stands for Rhesus Hominid Negative and Rhesus blood factor or "D" antigen absent. If RhD is present, you are RhD positive for the Rhesus blood factor and the "D" antigen is present on your red blood cells. Rhesus positive means a common ancestral gene can be traced back to the Rhesus monkey. Science has not determined the source or origin of Rh negative blood. Nearly 85% of all human beings have

Rh-positive blood, though it varies by ethnicity, while only 15% of the entire global population is known to have the RH negative blood factor. This factor is independent of the A, B, AB, and O blood groups most people are familiar with. There are four main blood groups.

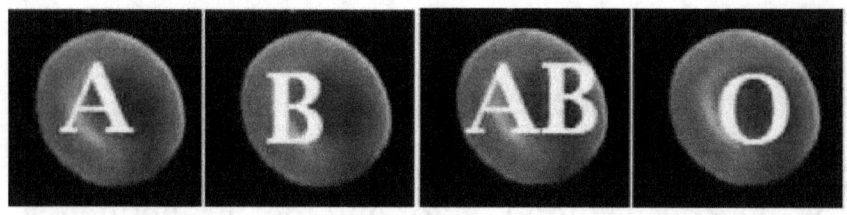

The Rh system is more complicated than the ABO system, because of the many different positive and negative possibilities that could be inherited. Rh negative is recessive and requires two negatives to be expressed.

Mother's Rh Type	Father's Rh Type	Possible Baby Rh Type
+ / +	+ / +	+ / +
+ / −	+ / +	+ / + + / −
+ / −	+ / −	+ / + + / − − / −
+ / −	− / −	+ / − − / −
− / −	+ / −	+ / − − / −
− / −	− / −	− / −

Blood type O is the most common of the blood groups. O RhD negative is the most unique of the blood types. It is the universal blood donor, makes up less than 7% of the global population and this extraordinary blood that can save lives of any other blood type. O negative can donate blood to all blood types, positive or negative but blood type except another O negative donor cannot receive blood from any other.

27

		Donor							
	Type	O-	O+	B-	B+	A-	A+	AB-	AB+
R **e** **c** **i** **p** **i** **e** **n** **t**	AB+	●	●	●	●	●	●	●	●
	AB-	●		●		●		●	
	A+	●	●			●	●		
	A-	●				●			
	B+	●	●	●	●				
	B-	●		●					
	O+	●	●						
	O-	●							

Attempts at creating RhD negative synthetic blood have not been successful. The protein in Rh positive blood can be cloned, that of Rh negative blood cannot.

Frequency

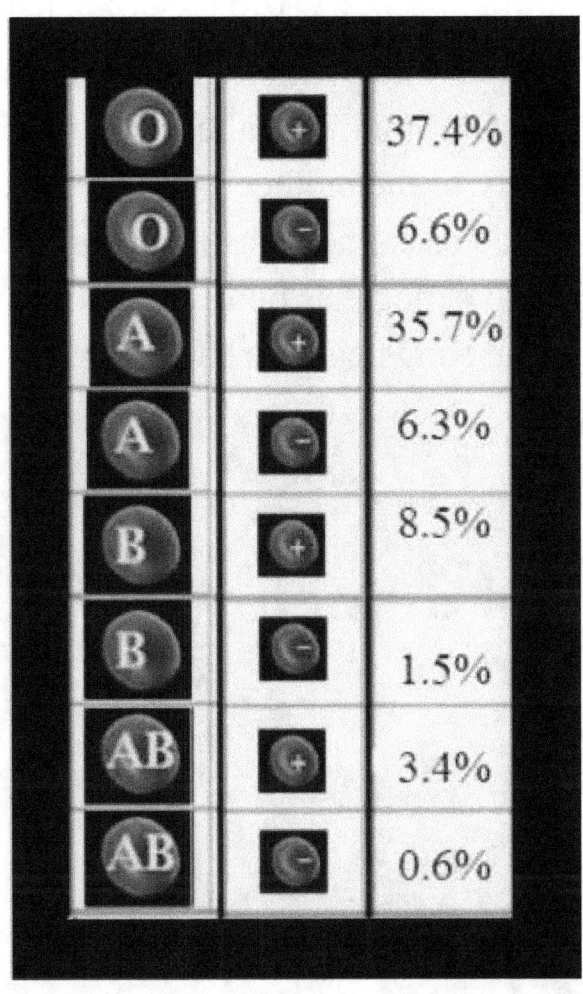

A Rh-negative pregnant mother's body will develop antibodies to her RhD positive baby without medical intervention of, "RhoGam" Rho (D) Immune Globulin. The allergic reaction due to the inability of the mother's body to recognize the Rhesus factor is known as Hemolytic Disease. A RhD positive mother's body does not develop antibodies the RhD negative baby.

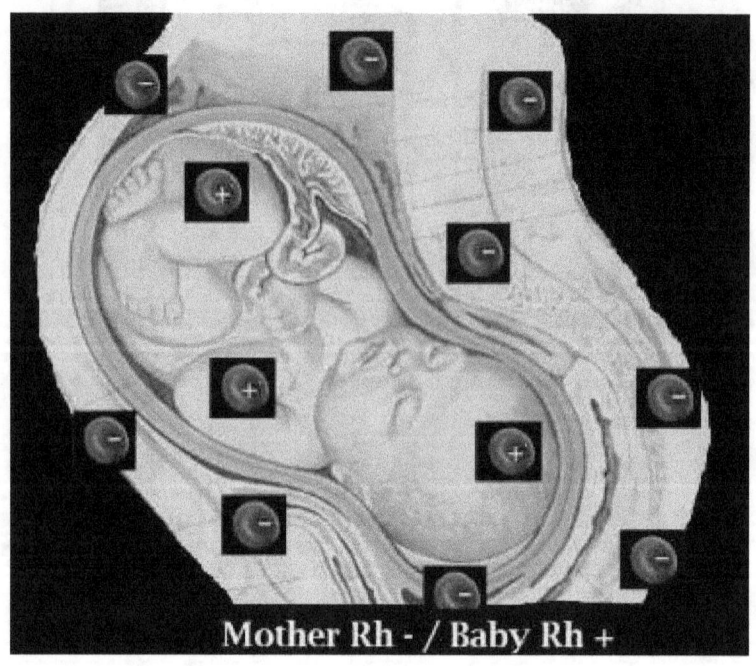

Mother Rh - / Baby Rh +

CHAPTER 3
HISTORY OF DISCOVERY 1930'S

1937 RHD NEGATIVE

Karl Landsteiner and Alexander S. Wiener German scientist discovered the Rh factor in 1937 (named after the Rhesus monkeys used as test subjects), while researching problems in blood transfusions. The A, B.O blood group systems were discovered by Karl Landsteiner in 1901. Before the invention of RhoGam, Dr. Wiener created the first medical procedure to treat the problem associated with Rh negative mother's carrying Rh positive babies.

A complete blood transfusion for the affected baby was performed, and many lives were saved. It was considered extremely rare.

1938 CATAMENIAL ENDOMETRIOSIS IN THE CHEST

The first reported cases of Catamenial Endometriosis in the chest were in the 1930's. Menstrual bleeding from a lung tumor associated with endometriosis was by Schwarz in 1938. A laboratory investigation by Hobbs and Bortnick in 1940 was able to produce pulmonary endometriosis in rabbits by intravenous infusion of endometrial tissue suspension.

Bungeler and associates in 1939 reported findings of three small nodules of endometriosis on the right upper pleural surface in a 42-year-old woman. Nicholson in 1951 was the first to report histologically proven endometriosis in a clinical case of recurrent hemorrhagic pleural effusion.

Many cases of endometriosis have been reported within the thorax in various sites: lung parenchyma, pleura, diaphragm, myocardium and bronchial tree. It has been referred to as Thoracic, Pulmonary, Extra-pelvic, Ectopic and Lung Endometriosis. Catamenial endometriosis in the chest was considered extremely rare but actually continues to be, under recognized and under diagnosed.

OXYGEN (O2) CONNECTION AND CO2

CELLULAR RESPIRATION

The body attempts to adjust to lower oxygen environments, by stimulating the heart and lungs to increase their functions and even over the long term, to increase in size. Blood vessels dilate and new capillaries are formed in the heart, brain and skeletal muscles. Other blood factors increase like hemoglobin, myoglobin, etc., to make the blood capable of carrying more oxygen and on a cellular level there is a growth of the cellular structures needed for the metabolism of oxygen

RhD protein plays a significant role as a channel for CO2 gas (carbon dioxide) across cell membranes in the body: "Rh proteins act as gas channels that help speed the transfer of carbon dioxide (CO2) in and out of red blood cells. Rh (Rhesus) proteins are CO2 channels. RhD is to help maintain the flexible, flattened shape of the red cell

WHILE IN THE AF STATIONED IN OSAN, SOUTH KOREA A CATAMENIAL PNEUMOTHORAX OCCURRED RESULTING IN THE PLACEMENT OF TWO CHEST TUBES. THE HOSPITAL IN OSAN DIDN'T HAVE CAT SCAN CAPABILITIES, SO I WAS TAKEN BY AMBULANCE TO YONGSON ARMY HOSPITAL, APPROXIMATELY ONE HOUR AWAY. THE BUMPY RIDE WITH TWO CHEST TUBES IN PLACE AND A PORTABLE SUCTION UNIT WOULD PROVE TO BE AN UNEXPLAINABLE EVENT COMMONLY REFERRED TO AS A MIRACLE. THE RIDE TO THE HOSPITAL WAS FAIRLY INSIGNIFICANT EXCEPT FOR THE MALFUNCTION OF THE PORTABLE SUCTION ATTACHED TO THE CHEST TUBE. I ARRIVED AT YONGSON HOSPITAL SAFELY AND SUCCESSFULLY COMPLETED THE CAT SCAN PROCEDURE.

DURING THE DRIVE HOME IT STARTED TO SNOW QUICKLY BECOMING AN INTENSE WINTER STORM CAUSING WHITE OUT EMERGENCY ROAD CONDITIONS. THE BLIZZARD PROMPTED LAW ENFORCEMENT TO CLOSE THE ROADS TO ALL EXCEPT EMERGENCY VEHICLES AND THEY COULD TRAVEL NO FASTER THAN 5 – 10 MPH DUE TO ZERO VISIBILITY. THE MEDICAL TECHNICIAN AND I BEGAN TO HEAR A STRANGE NOISE LIKE I WAS BREATHING IN A BARREL OR HOLE, AND I WAS BECOMING PROGRESSIVELY SHORT OF BREATH WHILE TRYING TO YELL FOR THE TECHNICIAN TO CALL MY DOCTOR AND TELL HIM TO BE WAITING BECAUSE I COULD NOT BREATHE.

WE ARRIVED AT THE HOSPITAL THREE HOURS LATER, AND TEAM DISCOVERED ONE OF THE CHEST TUBES PARTIALLY DISCONNECTED. THE TERRIBLE NOISE WE HEARD IN THE AMBULANCE WAS AIR TRAPPED IN THE MUSCLE AS MY LUNG COLLAPSED MORE AND MORE DUE TO THE ONE-WAY VALVE ON THE LOWER CHEST TUBE DISLODGING. I WAS FORTUNATE TO BE ALIVE.

Did my O RhD negative blood, oxygen (O2), carbon dioxide (CO2) cellular respiration facilitation protect me while trapped? The only time my O2 has ever dropped was during a tension pneumothorax; it remained 98 to 100 mm Hg on room air during all other Catamenial Pneumothoraces

CHAPTER 4
THEORIES

CATAMENIAL ECTOPIC ENDOMETRIOSIS

Many theories have been proposed to explain catamenial ectopic endometriosis in distant organs and now in males. To date, all the theories remain inconclusive.

Sampson's Theory- suggests that during a woman's menstrual cycle, retrograde flow of sloughed endometrial cells flow backward through the fallopian tubes into the pelvic cavity where endometrial cells can invade other body tissue.

Meyer's Theory- coelomic metaplasia, cells can change from one type to another but arise from the same embryologic origin or precursor. (Undifferentiated cells of the peritoneal surface differentiate into endometrial cells). *MOST PROBABLE FOR MEN*

Halban's Theory- vascular lymph transmission suggests that endometrial cells flow through vascular or lymphatic channels to enter other organs.

RHESUS D NEGATIVE

The source of RhD negative blood has not been located prompting some to theorize it did not originate on earth. Ancient text from Sumerian tablets is quite revealing.

Science has proposed a theory of random mutation for adaptation.

An article titled ABO and Rhesus blood groups and risk of endometriosis in a French Caucasian population of 633 patients living in the same geographic area, concludes "Rh-negative women are twice as likely to develop endometriosis" (see references)

Rh negative status referred to as Copper Based Aquatic Blood and in China as panda blood is studied around the world.

A list of Rh negative traits noticed throughout generations has been analyzed and compiled.

Empathetic Illnesses - senses and feels the pains of others

Photophobia - sensitive to bright light

Food allergies

Low blood pressure

Slow heart rate

Low body temperature

Hypothyroid

Different eye color

Piercing eyes

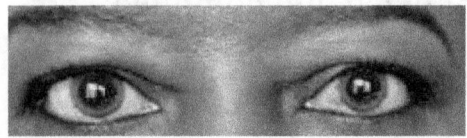

Healers

Blood cannot be cloned

Increased senses – hearing, smell, vision

Increased psychic and ESP abilities

Intuition

Highly electrical – disrupts electrical devices

Experience unexplained phenomenon

Psychic dream ability

Extra vertebrae or rib

Higher magnetism around body

High sensitivity to electromagnetic fields.

Have an affinity for science and space

Truth seekers

Para-normal occurrences

Desire for higher wisdom

A sense of a 'mission' in life

Idiopathic and autoimmune illnesses
(endometriosis in distant organs would qualify)

Affinity for space and science

Interesting, I saw my life in many of these traits.

An extremely important revelation, the "Shroud of Turin revealed Jesus was AB negative".

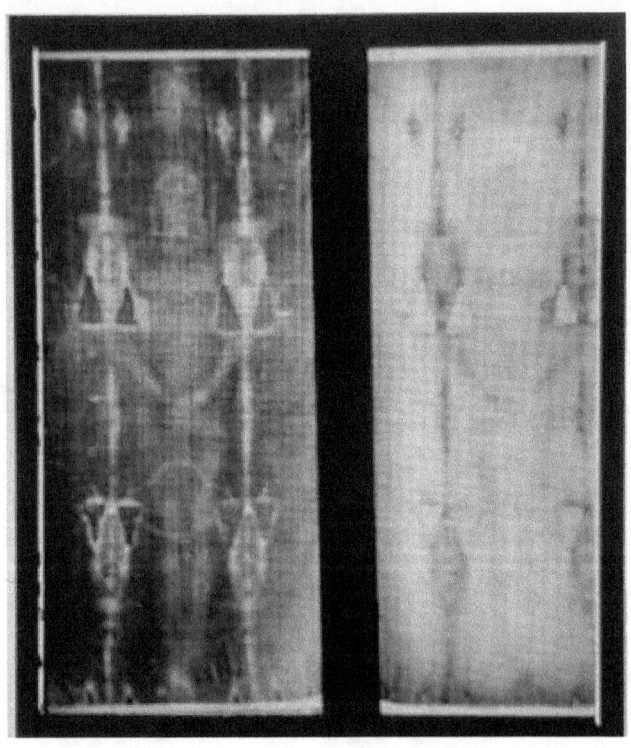

CHAPTER 5
FOODS TO AVOID

Foods to avoid became a frightening issue for me, so I set out to compare notes with other catamenial endometriosis sufferers. There are general recommendations for foods to avoid, like dairy, eggs, and gluten which cause inflammation, GI upset, mucous, irritation and other tolerable symptoms but nothing severe. For as long as I can remember, over 30 years, legumes cause a severe reaction producing gas and pressure in my chest.

Not a true allergy causing hive, rash or anaphylaxis, but pressure severe enough my chest lifts and I have to sleep at an angle or sitting up because it affects my breathing so severely. The other food is chocolate, after years of enjoyment, a true intolerance developed in 2009. This should have been welcomed to help me control weight.

After researching eating for blood type and knowing I was O negative from the military everything began to make sense. The sensitivity to tomatoes and potatoes classified as nightshades, a new welcomed term gave me the information I needed. It is so great to feel you are not alone.

REFERENCES

Roberts LM, Redan J, Reich H, **Extraperitioneal Endometriosis, Catamenial Pneumothoraces, And Review of the Literature.** JSLS. 2003 Oct-Dec;7(4):371-5.

Maurer ER, Schaal JA, Mendex Fl **Chronic recurring spontaneous Pneumothorax due to endometriosis of the diaphragm.** JAMA 1958: 168: 2013-2014

Avent ND, Reid ME.**The Rh blood group system: a review**. Blood. 2000;95:375–87

Matalliotakis I, Cakmak H, Goumenou A, Sifakis S, Ziogos E, Arici A. **ABO and Rh blood groups distribution in patients with endometriosis.** Archives of Gynecology and Obstetrics. 2009;280(6):917–919.

Borghese B, Chartier M, Souza C, Santulli P, Lafay-Pillet MC, de Ziegler D, Chapron C. **ABO and Rhesus Blood Groups and Risk of Endometriosis in a French Caucasian Population of 633 Patients Living in the Same Geographic Area** Biomed Res Int. 2014; 2014: 618964. Published online 2014 August 27. doi: 10.1155/2014/618964 PMCID: PMC4160609

Ngô C, Chéreau C, Nicco C, Weill B, Chapron C, Batteux F. **Reactive oxygen species controls endometriosis progression.** The American Journal of Pathology. 2009;175(1):225–234.

Kustu S1, Inwood W. **Biological gas channels for NH3 and CO2: evidence that Rh (Rhesus) proteins are CO2 channels.** Transfus Clin Biol. 2006 Mar-Apr;13(1-2):103-10. Epub 2006 Mar 24.

Dean L. **Blood Groups and Red Cell Antigens** [Internet]. Bethesda (MD): National Center for Biotechnology Information (US); 2005.

Bruce LJ. **Red cell membrane transport abnormalities.** Curr Opin Hematol. 2008 May;15(3):184-90. doi: 1097/MOH.0b013e3282f97b0a.

Landsteiner K and Wiener AS. **An agglutinable factor in human blood recognized by immune sera for rhesus blood.** Proc Soc Exp Biol Med, 1940, 43: 223-22

Schwartz, O. H.: **Endometriosis of the Lung.** In discussion of "Endometriosis, a Clinical and Surgical Review" by V. S. Counsellor, Am. J. Obst. & Gynec. 36: 887, 1938

Hobbs, J. E., and Bortnick, A. R.: **Endometriosis of Lungs: Experimental and Clinical** Study, Am. J. Obst. & Gynec. 40: 832 1940.

Charles, D.: **Endometriosis and Hemorrhagic Pleural Effusion,** Obst. & Gynec. 10: 309. 1957

Lattes, R., Shepard, F., Tovell, H., and Wylie, R.: **Clinical and Pathological Study of Endo-metriosis of Lung**, Surg., Gynec. & Obst. 103:552, 1956

Oliker AJ, Harris AE. **Endometriosis of the bladder in a male patient.**J Urol. 1971 Dec;106(6):858-9.

Schrodt GR, Alcorn MO, Ibanez J. **Endometriosis of the male urinary system**: a case report. J Urol. 1980 Nov;124(5):722-3.

González RS, Vnencak-Jones CL, Shi C, Fadare O. **Endomyometriosis ("Uterus-like mass") in an XY Male**: Case Report With Molecular Confirmation and Literature Review. Int J Surg Pathol. 2014 Aug;22(5):421-6. doi: 10.1177/1066896913501385. Epub 2014 Mar 19.

Martin JD Jr, Hauck AE. **Endometriosis in the male**. Am Surg. 1985 Jul;51(7):426-3

Fukunaga M **Paratesticular endometriosis in a man with a prolonged hormonal therapy for prostatic carcinoma.** Pathol Res Pract. 2012 Jan 15;208(1):59-61. doi: 10.1016/j.prp.2011.10.007. Epub 2011 Nov 21.

Jabr FI1, Mani V2. **An unusual cause of abdominal pain in a male patient: Endometriosis.** Avicenna J Med. 2014 Oct;4(4):99-101. doi: 10.4103/2231-0770.140660

Beckman EN, Pintado SO, Leonard GL, Sternberg WH. **Endometriosis of the prostate.** Am J Surg Pathol 1985;9:3.74-9

Jason L Nelles, Wen-Yang Hu, and Gail S Prins,† **Estrogen action and prostate cancer.** Expert Rev Endocrinol Metab. 2011 May; 6(3): 437–451.

Zugor V1, Krot D, Rösch WH, Schrott KM, Schott GE. **Endometriosis of the ureter and urinary bladder.** Urologe A. 2007 Jan;46(1):71-8; quiz 79.

Simona Sacco,corresponding author Silvia Ricci, Diana Degan, and Antonio Carolei. **Migraine in women: the role of hormones and their impact on vascular diseases.** J Headache Pain. 2012 Apr; 13(3): 177–189.

Doodipala Samba Reddy **Neuroendocrine aspects of catamenial epilepsy.** Horm Behav. 2013 Feb; 63(2): 254–266.

Silberstein SD **Headache and female hormones: what you need to know**. Curr Opin Neurol. 2001 Jun;14(3):323-33.

Witte A1, Guilbaud O. **Endometriosis of the diaphragm.** Diagnostic aspects apropos of a case without pneumothorax. Rev Med Interne. 1995;16(7):527-32.

Ho VH1, Wilson MW, Linder JS, Fleming JC, Haik BG. **Bloody tears of unknown cause: case series and review of the literature**. Ophthal Plast Reconstr Surg. 2004 Nov;20(6):442-7.

Türkçüoğlu I1, Türkçüoğlu P, Kurt J, Yildirim H. **Presumed nasolacrimal endometriosis**. Ophthal Plast Reconstr Surg. 2008 Jan-Feb;24(1):47-8. doi: 10.1097/IOP.0b013e31815c9053.

Brekken AL, Massey FM **A common adnexal mass in an uncommon patient**: a case report. J Reprod Med. 1980 Oct;25(4):171-2.

Nötzold A, Moubayed P, Sievers HH. **Endometriosis in the thoracic aorta.** N Engl J Med. 1998 Oct 1;339(14):1002-3.

Flyckt R1, Lyden S, Roma A, Falcone T. **Post-menopausal endometriosis with inferior vena cava invasion requiring surgical management.** Hum Reprod. 2011 Oct;26(10):2709-12. doi: 10.1093/humrep/der260. Epub 2011 Aug 10

Nasu K1, Narahara H, Hayata T, Miyakawa I, Takahashi S, Fukunaga Y, Nomura Y. **Ureteral obstruction caused by endometriosis.** Gynecol Obstet Invest. 1995;40(3):215-6.

Cheng CH, Kuo HC, Su B. **Endometriosis in a kidney with focal xanthogranulomatous pyelonephritis and a perinephric abscess.** BMC Res Notes. 2015 Oct 21;8:591. doi: 10.1186/s13104-015-1574-1.

Hsu M, Terris B, Wu TT, Zen Y, Eng HL, Huang WT, Yeh MM. **Endometrial cysts within the liver: a rare entity and its differential diagnosis with mucinous cystic neoplasms of the liver.** Hum Pathol. 2014 Apr;45(4):761-7. doi: 10.1016/j.humpath.2013.11.005. Epub 2013 Nov 21.

Bouras AF1, Vincentelli A, Boleslawski E, Truant S, Liddo G, Prat A, Pruvot FR, Zerbib P. **Liver endometriosis presenting as a liver mass associated with high blood levels of tumoral biomarkers.** Clin Res Hepatol Gastroenterol. 2013 Jun;37(3):e85-8.

Liu K, Zhang W, Liu S, Dong B, Liu Y. **Hepatic endometriosis: a rare case and review of the literature.** Eur J Med Res. 2015 Apr 4;20:48. doi: 10.1186/s40001-015-0137-1.

Tuech JJ1, Rousselet MC, Boyer J, Descamps P, Arnaud JP, Ronceray J. **Endometrial cyst of the liver: case report and review**. Fertil Steril. 2003 May;79(5):1234-6

Laghzaoui O1, Laghzaoui M. **Nasal endometriosis: apropos of 1 case**. J Gynecol Obstet Biol Reprod (Paris). 2001 Dec;30(8):786-8.

Monrad-Hansen PW1, Buanes T, Young VS, Langebrekke A, Qvigstad E. **Endometriosis of the pancreas**. J Minim Invasive Gynecol. 2012 Jul-Aug;19(4):521-3. doi: 10.1016/j.jmig.2012.03.011.

Acar T, Acar N, Çelik SC, Ekinci N, Tarcan E, Çapkınoğlu E. **Endometriosis within the sigmoid colon/extragenital endometriosis.** Ulus Cerrahi Derg. 2015 Jul 10;31(4):250-2. doi: 10.5152/UCD.2015.2770. eCollection 2015.

Sanchez Cifuentes A, Candel Arenas MF, Albarracín Marín-Blázquez A. **Intestinal endometriosis. Our experience.** Rev Esp Enferm Dig. 2016 Mar 29;108. doi: 10.17235/reed.2016.4292/2016.

Baker GS, Parsons WR, Welch JS.
Endometriosis within the sheath of the sciatic nerve. Report of two patients with progressive paralysis. J Neurosurg. 1966 Dec;25(6):652-5.

Ceccaroni M1, Clarizia R, Cosma S, Pesci A, Pontrelli G, Minelli L. **Cyclic sciatica in a patient with deep monolateral endometriosis infiltrating the right sciatic nerve.** J Spinal Disord Tech. 2011 Oct;24(7):474-8. doi: 10.1097/BSD.0b013e31820fc53b.

Steck WD, Helwig EB. **Cutaneous endometriosis**. JAMA 1965;191:101-4.

Beischer NO. **Endometriosis of an episiotomy scar cured by pregnancy.** Obstet Gynecol 1966; 28:15-21.

Dhawan AK1, Singh S, Tyagi M, Arora V. **Scar with recurrent serosanguinous discharge.** Clin Exp Dermatol. 2015 Mar;40(2):213-5. doi: 10.1111/ced.12462. Epub 2014 Sep 23.

ABOUT THE AUTHOR

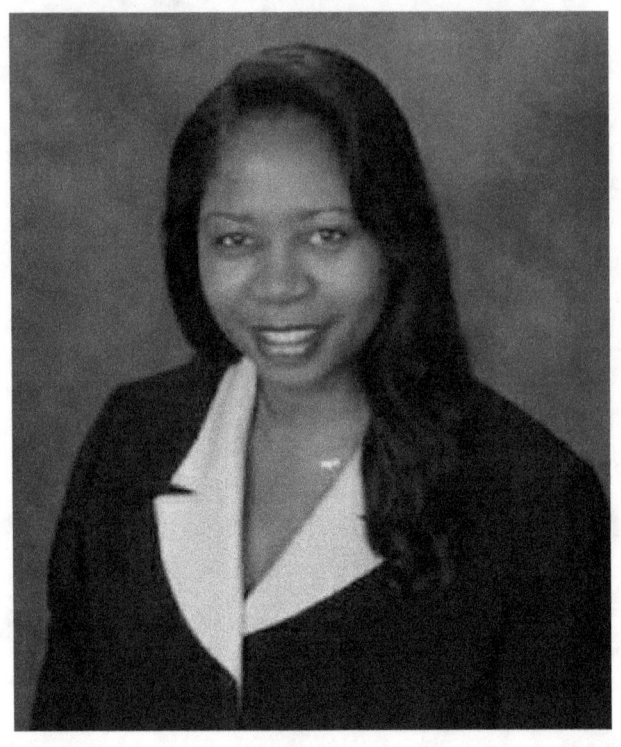

DR. GLYNIS D. WALLACE, A GRADUATE OF TUFTS UNIVERSITY SCHOOL OF DENTAL MEDICINE, FORMER MAJOR IN THE USAF, INTERNATIONALLY KNOWN AUTHOR. DR. WALLACE CREATED THE WIKIPEDIA PAGE FOR CATAMENIAL PNEUMOTHORAX IN 2006 WHICH STIMULATED A MOVE TO ACTION WITH UNDETERMINED NUMBERS OF WOMEN BEING DIAGNOSED GLOBALLY WITH THORACIC ENDOMETRIOSIS SYNDROME.

OTHER BOOKS BY

DR. GLYNIS D. WALLACE

"Living With Lung and Colon Endometriosis: Catamenial Pneumothorax" (*First known book on*

Catamenial Pneumothorax (menstrual lung collapse)

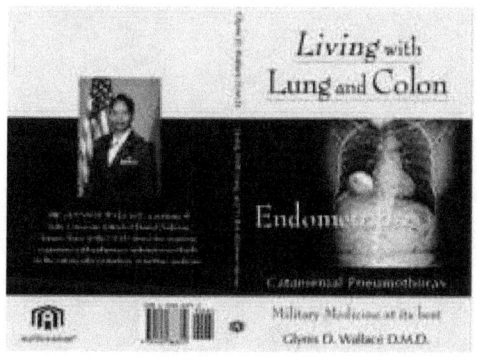

"Secrets of Faith: Catamenial Solutions"

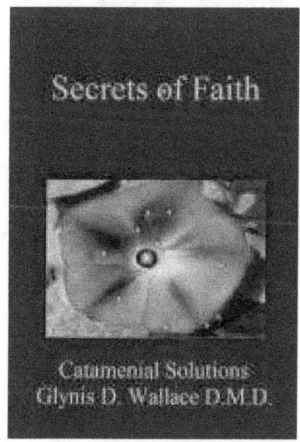

ONE LAST THING

If you liked this book, I would be very grateful if you would please leave a short review on Amazon.